GINGER

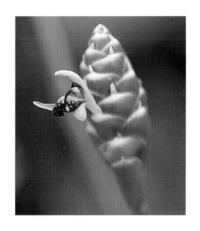

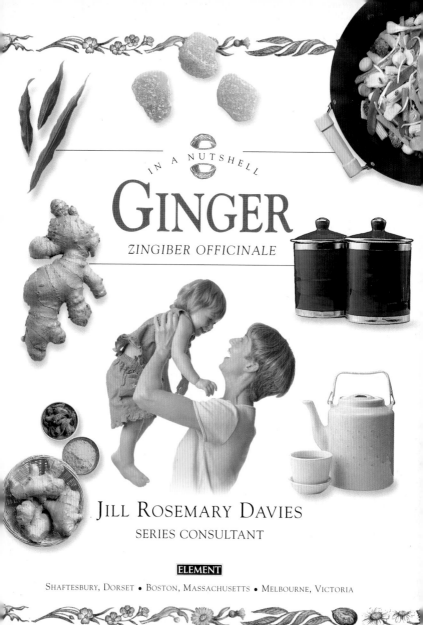

IN A NUTSHELL

GINGER

ZINGIBER OFFICINALE

JILL ROSEMARY DAVIES

SERIES CONSULTANT

ELEMENT

SHAFTESBURY, DORSET • BOSTON, MASSACHUSETTS • MELBOURNE, VICTORIA

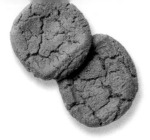

Series Consultant Jill Rosemary Davies
Text Dr. Joseph F. Ryan

First published in Great Britain in 2000 by
ELEMENT BOOKS LIMITED
Shaftesbury, Dorset SP7 8BP

Published in the USA in 2000 by
ELEMENT BOOKS INC.
160 North Washington Street,
Boston MA 02114

Published in Australia in 2000 by
ELEMENT BOOKS LIMITED
and distributed by
Penguin Australia Ltd.
487 Maroondah Highway,
Ringwood, Victoria 3134

For growing and harvesting, calendar
information applies only to the northern
hemisphere (US zones 5–9).

Designed and created for Element Books with
The Bridgewater Book Company Ltd.

ELEMENT BOOKS LIMITED
Editorial Director Sue Hook
Project Editor Kate John
Assistant Editor Annie Hamshaw-Thomas
Group Production Director Clare Armstrong
Production Controller Hannah Turner

THE BRIDGEWATER BOOK COMPANY
Art Director Terry Jeavons
Senior Designer Tony Seddon
Designer Jane Lanaway
Editorial Director Fiona Biggs
Project Editor Lorraine Turner
DTP Designer Trudi Valter
Photography Guy Ryecart
Illustrations Michael Courtney
Picture Research Liz Moore

Printed and bound in Portugal.

Library of Congress Cataloging
in Publication data is available

British Library Cataloguing
in Publication data is available

ISBN 1 86204 708 1

*The publishers wish to thank the following for
the use of pictures:* AKG London Ltd: 10r,
11b; Bridgeman Art Library: 11t, 12b, 13r,
22b; Bruce Coleman Collection: 24b; Eye
Ubiquitous: 8t, 28t; Garden Picture Library:
26; Image Bank: 43t; Science Photo
Library: 17b, 20t, 42t; Stokes Tropicals, 6b;
Tony Stone Images: 18, 20b, 49b, 51; Trip:
1, 27t, 28b, 29b.

The publishers also wish to thank: Professor
Peter Houghton, Kings College, London,
for technical information; the Wellcome
Trust, Patricia East, *and* Dorothy Ryan *for
research and support.*

Contents

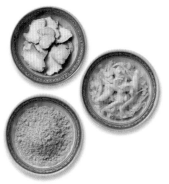

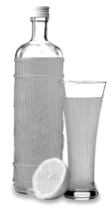

Introduction

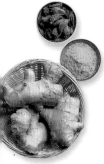

AN ANCIENT REMEDY, *Ginger is used for many purposes, most notably perhaps for nausea. As a stimulant, it helps to improve peripheral circulation. In fevers, it promotes perspiration. It is also excellent for treating dyspepsia, colic, and flatulence. Externally, it forms the base for various muscle strain and fibrositis treatments. Ginger, however, has many other uses and well deserves its worldwide reputation – gained over thousands of years – as a powerful aid for healing.*

ABOVE **Turmeric and Cardamom are related to Ginger.**

Ginger, which is used in a vast array of sweet and savory dishes around the world, is a tender, creeping perennial. It grows in tropical climates from underground rhizomes, which are commonly (but incorrectly) called "roots." The plant may reach 3–4ft (1–1.2m) in height. It has dark, erect stems that resemble bamboo, and lance-shaped leaves. The thick, fibrous, buff to white tuberous rhizome is perennial and has a spicy, warming smell and a pungent, citruslike taste. *Zingiber officinale* blooms have a small green inflorescence with white and maroon flowers. In other species, colors can range through to reds and oranges.

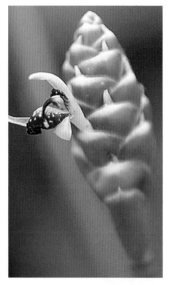

ABOVE **The orchidlike flower of Zingiber officinale, which blooms in tropical climates.**

The botanical name for Ginger – *Zingiber officinale* – was given by the Swedish botanist Linnaeus. It comes from the Sanskrit word *singabera*, which means "shaped like a horn." The term *officinale* simply means that the plant is commonly available and is useful to humans in medicine and as a food. Ginger is known as *Sheng jian* in Chinese, and has a number of English synonyms including Jamaican Ginger. The rhizome and essential oil are used medicinally.

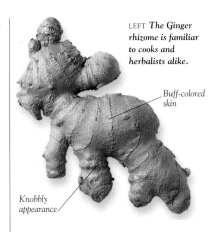

LEFT *The Ginger rhizome is familiar to cooks and herbalists alike.*

Buff-colored skin

Knobbly appearance

WHAT TO BUY

Always try to buy Ginger that has been certified as grown organically to ensure the best healing results. Because of its culinary uses, fresh and dried Ginger is widely available in supermarkets. Ginger is also obtainable in capsule or tincture form, or as an essential oil, in drug stores, health food and herbal stores, or by mail order.

DEFINITION

Botanical family: Ginger, or specifically *Zingiber officinale*, is just one of about 1,400 species in the *Zingiberaceae* family, which also includes Turmeric and Cardamom. The plant is a native of Asia, but is grown throughout the tropics and wherever there is a rich soil and a warm climate.

Species: Although various *Zingiber* species are used medicinally, none of them have the same powerful beneficial effects as those of *Zingiber officinale*. There are, however, many naturally occurring varieties of *Zingiber officinale* – approximately 50 in India alone. Differing growing conditions and cultivation techniques result in each variety having its own unique aroma and flavor. For instance, milder examples tend to be found in China, and more pungent ones in Africa.

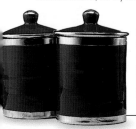

LEFT *Store Ginger in dark-glass jars to retain its healing properties.*

Exploring Ginger

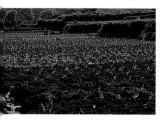

A NATIVE PLANT *of Asia, Ginger may be found throughout the tropics where it thrives in the warm climate and rich soils.*

LEFT **Fields of Ginger growing are a common sight in tropical parts of the world.**

WHERE TO FIND GINGER

Zingiber officinale is widespread throughout tropical regions. There are several theories as to where it originated; however, the most likely is that it came from Southeast Asia. Today, Ginger may be seen growing in China, India, Africa (notably in Nigeria and Sierra Leone), the West Indies (especially Jamaica), southern parts of the United States, and wherever the right soil and climate allow its growth.

COMMERCIAL GROWERS

Cultivation of Ginger in the United States is mainly confined to zone 9 – that is, to those regions on a latitude with Florida and southern Texas where the average annual minimum temperature is confined to between 20°–30°F (-7°–-1°C). It is widely cultivated in both the East and

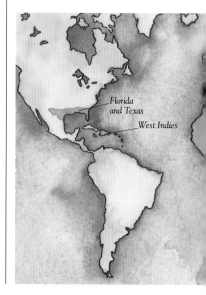

Florida and Texas

West Indies

West Indies, and some of the best-quality root is grown in Jamaica. Ginger is also cultivated commercially in China and Korea.

REQUIREMENTS FOR GROWTH

A rich, well-drained loam and light shade is needed for Ginger to grow well. In the wild, it thrives in the warm, humid conditions of the tropical forest floor, and the ideal temperature for its growth is in the region of 70–75°F (21–24°C). Although it is a tropical plant, Ginger can still be grown in cooler climates in greenhouses or conservatories. In the spring and summer, a heated greenhouse that provides plenty of humidity and shade will soon have the plants flourishing in broad, spreading clumps.

Indoors, the atmosphere will probably be too dry, although a warm kitchen is likely to offer the best environment. It is doubtful, however, that the plant will flower under these circumstances, though it does in greenhouses from time to time, such as those in botanical gardens. If grown in pots, repot annually in the spring. When the largest practical pot size has been reached, divide the plant and start again.

Propagate the plant by dividing the rhizomes as growth begins in the spring. These should be planted just below the surface of the soil (which should be good-quality compost), in greenhouse beds or pots.

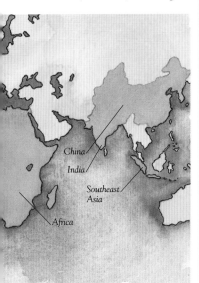

China

India

Southeast Asia

Africa

LEFT **As the map shows, Ginger grows in tropical regions across the world.**

RIGHT **A young Ginger plant grown in a greenhouse.**

A history of healing

VALUED SINCE *earliest times for its important healing properties, Ginger has enjoyed an excellent reputation in ancient Indian, traditional Chinese, and Western medicine. As a pungent spice and flavoring agent, Ginger also has an important place in the cuisine of countries all around the world.*

LEFT **The Chinese have known about Ginger's medicinal qualities for thousands of years.**

TRADITIONAL USES

Ginger has an ancient history. It is possible that as long as 5,000 years ago, spice caravans were carrying dried Ginger from India to the Middle East. Ginger is one of the best-known of spices, and it is believed that its medicinal properties have been known in China for thousands of years. Indeed, the plant was mentioned in Emperor Shen Hung's *Pen Tsao Ching* (*The Classic Book of Herbs*), which he wrote in 3000 BCE.

Although frequently associated with Traditional Chinese medicine, Ginger has an ancient reputation in India and is specifically mentioned in the

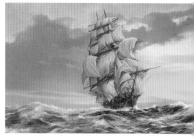

ABOVE **The Chinese have traded Ginger for millennia.**

Ayurveda, the Hindu manual of medicine written in the fifth century BCE. An ancient Indian proverb states: "Every good quality is contained in Ginger."

The ancient Greeks – such as Galen – knew and used Ginger. Inheriting the Greek traditions and knowledge, the ancient Romans also valued Ginger for its culinary and medicinal uses. For example, Largus (c.43 CE), a physician in the Roman army and the author of a book entitled *De*

Compositione Medicamentorum, described the Roman military expedition to Britain and was responsible for the introduction of Opium and Ginger to the island. Another Roman, Pedianos Dioscorides, wrote about Ginger in his famous *De Materia Medica* (77 CE). He was concerned to ensure a "better quality of drug" and mentioned, for example, some of the problems associated with the storage of Ginger.

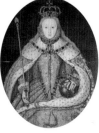

ABOVE **Queen Elizabeth I took Ginger to ward off indigestion.**

Subsequently, Ginger received a mention in the Islamic holy book, the *Koran*, where it says that among the righteous in Paradise "are passed vessels of silver and goblets of glass" and "a cup, the admixture of which is Ginger."

Later, when the spice came to medieval Europe, it was thought that it had come from the Garden of Eden. In the Middle Ages in England, just one pound of the spice was held to be equal in value to a sheep, and for a long time only the wealthy could afford to use it. Queen Elizabeth I used it as a digestive aid.

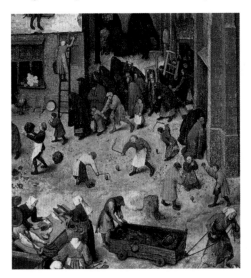

LEFT **To the ordinary people of medieval England, Ginger was a costly spice, well beyond their means.**

During the 15th century, a Spanish explorer called Francisco de Mendosa transplanted the Ginger plant and brought it back to Spain from the East Indies. Thereafter, following the arrival of Spanish explorers and settlers to the North American continent, Ginger was soon introduced and became naturalized there. British herbalist John Gerard wrote:

"Ginger, as Dioscorides reporteth, is right good with meat in sauces or otherwise in conditures; for it is of an heating and digesting qualitie."

RECENT HISTORY

Today, nothing has changed and fresh Ginger remains a key ingredient in many Asian dishes.

Ground Ginger helps to provide a spicy, warming flavor in cakes and cookies, as well as in ales,

BELOW **Ginger came to North America with the Spanish explorers.**

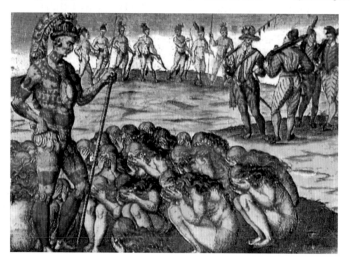

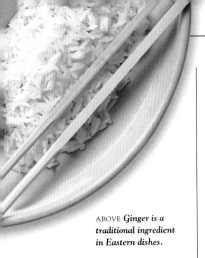

ABOVE *Ginger is a traditional ingredient in Eastern dishes.*

Traditionally, Ginger has also been added to many other remedies that rely on a mixture of herbs because it tends to reduce toxicity and side effects. As such, it is therefore of particular benefit when used in herbal combinations.

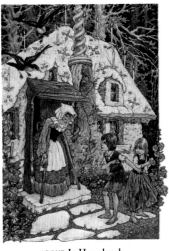

ABOVE **In** Hansel and Gretel, *children are enticed into a Gingerbread house.*

beers, and wine. Its familiar taste is part of our folklore. For example, the Gingerbread house in the tale *Hansel and Gretel* proved irresistible to children. Ginger has also been used to scent pomanders and potpourris.

As a very warming plant, Ginger is still held to be of particular value in the treatment of certain conditions. For example, it is ideal for people suffering from colds and chills, and as a circulatory stimulant. It promotes cleansing of the system through perspiration and reduces flatulence. Furthermore, it helps to alleviate nausea and, therefore, is an excellent remedy for motion sickness and morning sickness in pregnancy.

CAUTION

Ginger is contraindicated (not advised) in certain conditions. For example, it can irritate gastric ulcers. It can also aggravate hepatitis (see page 21) and some conditions of the kidney that involve inflammation (see page 42).

Anatomy of Ginger

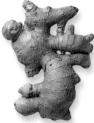

ABOVE *Ginger's "hand and fingers."*

IT IS THE ROOT of Ginger that provides the healing properties of the plant. Chemical analysis shows many substances in the root are responsible for helping to provide the herb's beneficial effects.

Fresh Ginger root is bulbous and fleshy. In the spice trade, the whole main segment is termed a "hand," and the branches that come from it are called "fingers." This is very apt, because fresh Ginger often resembles a hand with blunt, stubby fingers. The branching rhizome of Ginger is fleshy, full, and a little flattened in appearance; in taste it is fragrant and pungent.

Zingiber officinale occurs naturally in many different varieties – fifty can be found in India alone. Each variety has its own individual flavor and aroma.

LEFT **Rubbing Ginger ointment into the calf relieves cramp.**

Chemical constituents

Ginger is known to contain volatile oils (including borneol, camphene, citral, eucalyptol, linalol, phellandrene, zingiberine, and zingiberol), phenols (gingerol, zingerone, and shogaol), and resin.

The famous American herbalist Michael Tierra describes Ginger as "spicy, warm, and mainly affecting the lungs and stomach."

Some of Ginger's medicinal properties are contained in the chemicals responsible for its taste, the most noteworthy being gingerol and shogaol. The fragrance of Ginger is due to the volatile oil, which is composed of about 200 chemical substances and accounts for approximately 1–2.5% of the rhizome. Nutrients include carbohydrates, lipids, proteins, minerals, and vitamins. Among these may be found phosphorus, potassium, riboflavin, and vitamin C. Finally, synergists include zingibain, a protein-digesting enzyme that is known to act in a similar manner to bromelain in pineapple, and capsaicin, limonene, and curcumin. The latter is the main active constituent in Turmeric, which is closely related to Ginger.

It is clear that Ginger contains a vast and complex array of chemicals that, in combination, provide a powerful aid to healing. For example, the enzyme zingibain is believed to improve digestion as well as kill parasites and their eggs. Furthermore, zingibain enhances antibacterial and anti-inflammatory actions, and is thought to assist other anti-bacterials, such as antibiotics, by up to 50%. Ginger's ability to reduce inflammation is due to its

LEFT **Ginger may be sliced, shredded, or powdered for use in cooking and healing.**

Shredded Ginger

Sliced Ginger

Powdered Ginger

neutralizing action upon free radicals (see page 57), which are known to contribute to the problem. Finally, Ginger contains over 12 antioxidant constituents, the combined actions of which have been regarded as being more powerful than vitamin C.

SHELF LIFE OF ROOT
The fresh root can last up to two months in a refrigerator or cool larder; dried, powdered, or shredded root lasts up to one year; dried whole root lasts for 1–2 years. With suitable storage facilities, Ginger can last much longer, although the active constituents, especially the volatile oils, will gradually decrease with time.

Ginger in action

GINGER IS A REMARKABLE *remedy with a wide range of actions that are suitable for men, women, and children. It is very safe and has a record of use that stretches back thousands of years, across many cultures and continents.*

LEFT **The whole family can benefit from Ginger.**

HOW GINGER CAN HELP

Ginger promotes gastric secretion and is excellent for many kinds of digestive complaints, including indigestion, colic, and wind.

It is highly effective in combating nausea – whether due to pregnancy, travel, or following an anesthetic.

Ginger stimulates the circulation and is therefore beneficial for circulatory complaints including poor blood supply to the hands and feet, and for chilblains.

RIGHT **Warming Ginger tea wards off morning sickness.**

In fevers, Ginger is able to induce sweating, thereby helping to reduce body temperature.

It acts as a warming expectorant to encourage productive coughing and relieves sore throats when used as a gargle.

Ginger has antiseptic and antiparasitic effects: it is useful for bacterial infections in the digestive tract.

When used externally, it has an anti-inflammatory action and is a useful base in many preparations for treating muscle strains, joint sprains, and muscle pain.

HOW GINGER AFFECTS THE BODY

Many of the body's systems are affected by chemical constituents found in *Zingiber officinale*. Indeed, so complex are the actions of Ginger that it is almost impossible to list all its effects upon the body.

Ginger acts on the musculo-skeletal system in a similar way to aspirin, reducing the number of inflammatory factors, but without the side effects common to such anti-inflammatory drugs. As such, it has an important role to play in inflammatory disorders such as arthritis. In the digestive system, Ginger inhibits the growth of toxic microorganisms while simultaneously allowing beneficial bacteria to grow.

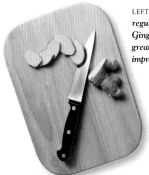

LEFT *Cooking regularly with Ginger is a great way to improve health.*

Ginger has an important effect upon the circulatory system too, helping to prevent the stagnation and congestion that can cause pain and disease. Arteries can become obstructed by the action of thromboxanes, which cause blood platelets to aggregate, eventually forming blood clots. This can lead to heart attacks and strokes. Ginger has now been found to be as effective as aspirin in reducing the formation of clots and subsequent blockages (see page 18). Research indicates that Ginger may strengthen the heart and lower blood cholesterol levels.

LEFT *Ginger can help to prevent blood cells from clotting in the arteries.*

MAIN EFFECTS

Ginger has a number of beneficial effects. However, the following properties are of particular use for therapeutic purposes:

Antispasmodic: It relaxes all types of muscle.

Aromatic: Ginger's aroma, flavor, and warmth help to stimulate the digestive system.

Carminative: The volatile oils in Ginger relax the stomach and stimulate peristalsis (the wavelike motion of food through the gut) thereby supporting digestion and reducing gas.

Diaphoretic: It induces perspiration and the elimination of toxins through the skin.

Rubefacient: Applied to the skin, Ginger stimulates and dilates the blood capillaries, increasing circulation.

Sialagogue: It promotes the secretion of saliva.

Stimulant: As a circulatory aid, it supports and speeds up the body's physiological systems.

ABOVE *An ultrasound scan showing a four-chamber view of the heart.*

GINGER AND HEART DISEASE

Of particular interest is Ginger's impact on the heart and circulation. As described on page 17, heart attacks and strokes are mainly caused by the obstruction of arteries supplying cardiac muscle and the brain. Obstructions occur due to the formation of clots via the "cascade effect" (see page 56). Ginger helps prevent this process from occurring by inhibiting various steps of the clot-forming cascade effect, which are under the influence of thromboxanes.

In 1980, researchers at Cornell Medical School in the United States reported that Ginger was as effective as aspirin in preventing clot formation. Since then, a number of studies have confirmed the beneficial effect Ginger has on the cardiovascular system.

RIGHT *Ginger treats the major systems of the body.*

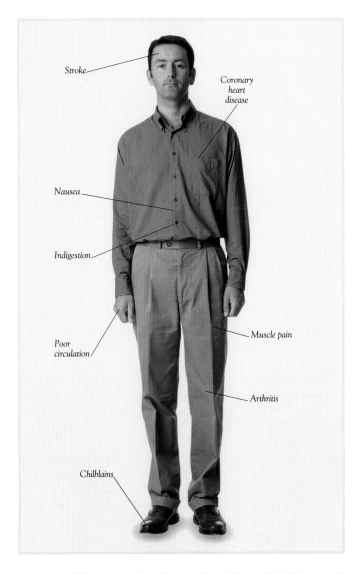

Stroke

Coronary
heart
disease

Nausea

Indigestion

Poor
circulation

Muscle pain

Arthritis

Chilblains

PROVEN RESULTS

Despite Ginger's long history of usage, medical studies of Ginger's effectiveness are limited. Some scientific studies, however, have been conducted, and a number of interesting findings have emerged.

⚘ *Zingiber officinale* has a powerful molluscicidal and antischistosomal effect, so is useful for treating schistosomiasis (blood fluke or bilharzia) infection, which is common in many countries without a treated water supply (Adewunmi, 1990).

⚘ One of Ginger's constituents, gingerol, is known to help blood circulation because it has an anticlotting or antiplatelet action due to its inhibition of thromboxane formation (Guh, 1995) (see page 17). It may, therefore, have an important role to play in the prevention of heart attacks and strokes.

⚘ An ethanol extract of Ginger has been shown to have antitumor effects on the skin of mice (Katiyar, 1996). Further research now needs to be undertaken to discover whether Ginger has a role to play in the prevention and treatment of skin cancer in humans.

BELOW *Bilharzia is a hazard when people drink untreated water, as is often the case in Third World countries.*

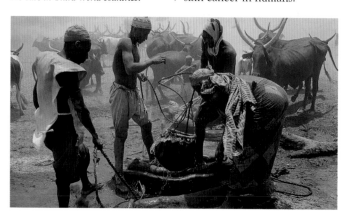

WHEN TO AVOID GINGER

As with other plant-based medications, it is best to confirm with your herbalist that it is safe to use Ginger in pregnancy. This is important because Ginger affects the endocrine (hormone) and reproductive systems. At least one German authority has said that it should not be taken at all in pregnancy, while some herbalists have suggested taking reduced amounts.

VE A false-color gamma *nera scan showing an* *ction in the right kidney.*

There is no known toxicity associated with ingesting Ginger. For those sensitive to it, however, it is best taken with food. Do not take Ginger if you have hepatitis – it can aggravate the condition. Also, consult a herbalist if you have any other liver complaint or kidney condition. Paradoxically, Ginger can be invaluable in some kidney and liver disorders and during pregnancy. Some specialists suggest that it should be avoided by people with gastric or peptic ulcers because it promotes gastric secretion.

ALLERGIC REACTION TO GINGER

There have been no reports of serious reactions to Ginger in the medical literature. As with almost any medication, there is a very small risk of a systemic (whole-body) allergic reaction (anaphylaxis). However, this is very rare and is more likely in people who already have an allergy to other plant extracts or herbal remedies. If someone does suffer a massive shock reaction to any substance, call an ambulance or immediately take the person to the nearest hospital accident and emergency department.

Reactions to Ginger are normally localized. Generally, they manifest themselves as contact dermatitis (a rash) where the extract has touched one specific part of the skin.

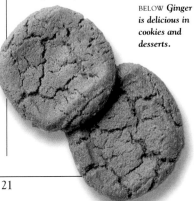

BELOW *Ginger is delicious in cookies and desserts.*

Energy and emotion

GINGER HAS MANY *powerful effects. Its complex chemistry produces a wide range of beneficial results for anyone who uses it regularly. Because Ginger stimulates the whole system, these positive results may include changes in a person's moods, emotions, and energy levels, with a consequent positive effect upon the mind and body.*

LEFT *Ginger improves health and vitality.*

Traditional Chinese and Ayurvedic (Indian) medicine seek to achieve harmony and health for the whole person, and aim to balance all aspects of an individual's body, mind, emotions, and spirit.

Traditional Chinese medicine categorizes Ginger as "pungent," signifying that it is able to warm the body and dispel cold. Associated with the element metal, which corresponds to the lungs in the Chinese system, Ginger expels toxins, opens the pores of the skin, and stimulates circulation. It is considered to be useful, therefore, for colds, influenza, mucus congestion, and fluid blockages in the body.

Ginger is a wonderful aid for helping the liver to rid itself of stored toxins, while overcoming any associated nausea or sickness. Over time, this has an effect on the emotions since detoxifying the liver can lift depressive, angry, or sad moods.

Ayurvedic and traditional Chinese medicine take a holistic view of

RIGHT *An engraving of Lord Brahma who revealed Ayurveda.*

lifestyle. Above all, physical exercise, good nutrition, and giving up bad habits such as smoking will create positive effects in the body, and lead to a general amelioration of existing illnesses and consequent enhancement of mood.

DIGESTION AND PLANT ENERGIES

One of Ginger's best-known effects is upon the digestive system. As a carminative, it helps to eliminate flatulence. It is also spasmolytic, helping to relax the intestinal muscles and soothe the digestive tract. It is also particularly effective at relieving nausea and sickness.

Ginger's energetic qualities reflect its uses. It is considered to be pungent, sweet, and warm. These qualities promote a tonic and supportive effect on the whole body and mind, inspiring a more outward-going, warm, and cheery outlook.

RIGHT *Ginger has an energizing, tonic effect on the whole family.*

ENERGY AND THE MIND

Ginger is such a powerful and safe healer that taking it inspires confidence. It is supportive of so many of the body's systems that its use helps to promote wide-ranging improvement. Its stimulant effects also help to give an overall energy boost to those who take it, which provides an extra benefit in addition to whatever localized influence it has upon specific parts of the body. Altogether, this provides a powerful lift to the mind and the emotions which, in turn, promote healing still further.

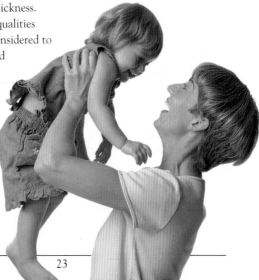

FLOWER REMEDIES

Flower remedies are a very subtle form of treatment. Ginger flower essence has a pulsating, vibrant gift, and is useful for those people who feel unconfident, dispirited, or unloved. It is a great healer of gloomy spirits and can help to lift depression. For people who are already in relative harmony in mind and body, it will further enliven them, both physically and mentally.

Zingiber officinale rarely blooms, and there will not be many occasions when this remedy can be prepared in countries outside the tropics, unless you grow this species in a heated greenhouse. However, flowers from any species of Ginger grown in other climates may be used to make a flower essence. It is worthwhile because this remedy imparts significant stimulation and balance to the body, thereby providing pure support.

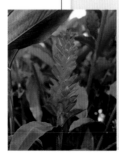

RIGHT **Another member of the Ginger family with red flowers found in Hawaii.**

TO MAKE A FLOWER ESSENCE

STANDARD QUANTITY
Approx. 1½ cups (350ml) each of spring water and brandy, and 3–4 Ginger flowers

1 Submerge freshly picked Ginger flowers in a glass bowl containing a small amount of spring water. Cover with clean, white cheesecloth and put in the sunshine for at least three hours. If the flowers wilt sooner, remove them earlier.

2 Use a twig to lift the flowers out of the bowl. Measure the remaining liquid, add an equal amount of brandy, then pour into sterilized dark glass bottles. Label clearly.

Recommended dosage
Adults: 4 drops under the tongue 4 times daily, or every ½ hour in times of crisis. Children: over 12 years, adult dose; 7–12 years, ½ adult dose; 1–7 years, ¼ adult dose; younger than 1 year, consult a qualified herbalist.

PLANT SPIRIT ENERGIES

The spirit of Ginger is not the same as its flower essence, which is solely connected with the flowering aspect of the plant. The spirit of Ginger enables the energy of the whole plant to be shared with us.

Ginger has been associated with love potions and other aphrodisiacs, and the purpose of the essence made from the entire

RIGHT *Yin and yang are harmonized in the Ginger plant.*

Ginger plant is to provide a balance between male and female qualities within both sexes – in terms of traditional Chinese medicine, this means helping to achieve harmony between the *yin* (female) and *yang* (male) energies. The flowers represent the female aspect of the plant, and the rhizome the male. When a good balance is achieved, over-aggressive tendencies are toned down and timid feelings corrected, whether appearing in men or women.

As well as its harmonizing qualities, Ginger's spirit offers warmth, calm, zest, and revitalization, all in a spirit of balance. It is therefore useful in a wide variety of situations.

CASE STUDY: HEART DISEASE

Jim never even suspected that he might suffer a heart attack. He was working very hard and felt that attending to his health would just have to wait a little longer. But he was wrong. He suddenly developed severe chest pains and even thought he was going to die. Luckily, prompt treatment in his local hospital saved him. To help prevent a further occurrence, his doctor told him to take aspirin on a regular basis. Jim, however, began to get stomach upsets and showed symptoms of a developing ulcer. His doctor, who was aware of the medical literature on the antiplatelet effect of gingerol, suggested Ginger as an alternative. Fortunately, Jim's stomach pains settled with this treatment, and the Ginger also helped to prevent any new clots from forming.

CAUTION

Ginger is a powerful healing remedy. Although it is useful in many conditions, it is an adjunct and not a replacement for professional expertise. In some cases, for example, Ginger may be more beneficial when used in combination with other treatments. It is important, therefore, to seek appropriate medical advice as necessary.

Growing, harvesting, and processing

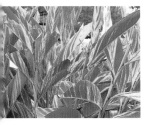

ALTHOUGH GINGER *is cultivated commercially in many tropical countries, and may readily be purchased in a range of stores, it can also be grown successfully in some gardens, under glass, or inside the home.*

LEFT **With the right conditions, Ginger flourishes as a cultivated crop.**

GROWING GINGER

Commercial Ginger grows best in loose, well-drained soil with a fairly high moisture-holding capacity. A pH of 5.5 to 6.5 is usually ideal.

The rhizome is prone to damage from burrowing worms, so the soil should be free from nematodes. It is also prone to bacterial damage (similar to that found on tomatoes). Commercially, non-organic crops are treated with relevant pesticides and herbicides.

Many rhizome types are used worldwide. Small ones produce pungent flavors and larger ones are less pungent but produce a greater yield.

Homegrown A fresh rhizome will produce new shoots quite rapidly if it is planted in moist compost in warm conditions – above 70°F (21°C). Ginger can even be propagated from a small piece of fresh root as long as it has one "eye" (similar to that found on potatoes) but preferably three or four.

Fill a small container with a good potting soil and plant the root on its side, parallel with the surface of the soil. The rhizome should be only just covered and the soil gently patted down over it. Allow a 1in (2½cm) gap

RIGHT **Plenty of rich soil is vital for growing Ginger.**

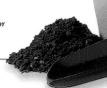

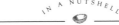
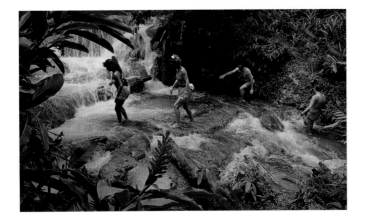

ABOVE *In the wild, Ginger grows abundantly in tropical rainforests.*

between the surface of the soil and the pot's rim for watering. Keep the pot in a warm place until green shoots emerge from the eye. You can then transplant into a larger pot filled with roughly equal amounts of loam and compost rich in organic matter and manure. Water this mixture regularly, and put a layer of mulch on top to prevent the upper layers of soil from drying out and the sensitive roots from being damaged. Ginger thrives in full sun but partial shade can

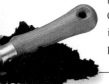

suffice. In warmer countries such as the Mediterranean, and even in milder climates such as the south of Britain, Ginger plants can remain outside all winter. In this way, large plants can become established and will flower each summer. However, in colder climates plants should be moved inside before the first frosts come. They can then be transferred outside in the spring.

When planting outdoors, place the Ginger plants in a raised bed about 10in (25cm) apart, and 4–6in (10–15cm) deep in the earth. Ginger tends to deplete soil of nutrients, so use a good mulch and renew it as necessary.

HARVESTING

Commercial The Ginger rhizome may be first harvested after approximately 8–10 months.

Early crops are sold commercially as fresh or "green" (at 6 months), or are used to produce Ginger pieces in syrup or crystallized Ginger. Otherwise Ginger is harvested after the leaves have died down (usually 8–10 months after planting) when the rhizome has fully matured. The internal flesh color should be pale yellow – any lateness in harvesting will reduce this colour and quality. Rhizomes are harvested in dry conditions, with a fork or cutlass to lift and break open the soil. They are then taken to a packhouse in field crates.

ABOVE
Crystallized Ginger is a delicacy.

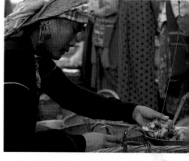

ABOVE *Ginger is an essential ingredient for meals in many parts of Asia.*

Homegrown Let the crop dry out during the last month before harvesting. Wait until the foliage has died down (usually 8–10 months from planting) then, using a fork, lift the mature rhizomes carefully from the soil. The longer they are left in the ground, the more fibrous and pungent they become.

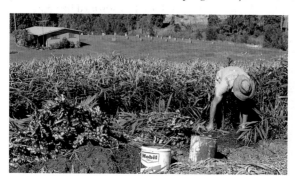

LEFT *Harvesting Ginger by hand is a hard, labor-intensive process.*

PROCESSING

Commercial After harvesting, the rhizomes are washed with a high-pressure hose before any mud has dried, taking care not to harm the delicate tissue that lies just below the skin's surface. This tissue contains many of the spice's valuable essential oils.

In India, rhizomes are sun-dried on clean floors for 7–10 days, and turned frequently. In America, they are dried quickly and then stored at 52°F (12°C), which keeps them fresh for 3 months. Mature Ginger, which is used to make dried Ginger, has a lower water content than the young "green Ginger." Ginger is often sold as a whole

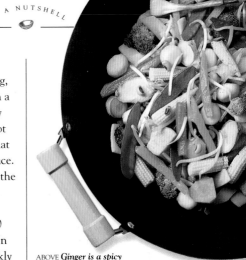

ABOVE *Ginger is a spicy addition to stir-fries and other dishes.*

root, but also ground or shredded for the culinary and medicinal markets.

Homegrown Fresh Ginger may be used at home in many ways. It must, of course, be cleaned in fresh water. Thereafter, it may be steamed, simmered, sautéed, boiled, or stir-fried like other root vegetables, as well as used medicinally.

To dry Ginger at home, put it in the oven for 2 hours at 100°F (38°C), or in the sun (minimum temperature 70°F/21°C) for at least 14 days. Ensure it is dried thoroughly before use.

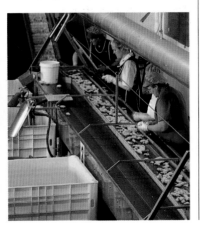

LEFT *Ginger is processed quickly and efficiently in factories.*

Preparations for internal use

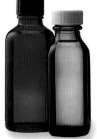

THERE ARE MANY WAYS *to take Ginger internally, using the fresh rhizome or dried powder. With either, look for fresh, well-colored forms that have a good taste and vibrancy about them. Cooking with Ginger regularly in sweet and savory dishes means that one benefits from its wide range of medicinal properties as well as enjoying its unique, spicy taste.*

LEFT **Tinctures are convenient medicines.**

TINCTURE

A tincture is made by soaking the chopped rhizome or powder in alcohol, which destroys bacteria and fungi. Subsequently the rhizome or powder is transferred to a mix of alcohol and water since some of Ginger's useful healing substances cannot survive long periods in high concentrations of alcohol.

Tinctures are convenient ways to take medicines. Freshly grated Ginger produces a medium-strength and balanced tincture while the powder creates one that is far stronger, both in terms of taste and some medicinal effects.

ESSENTIAL OIL

The essential oil is made by bubbling steam through a mash of Ginger. The highly concentrated essential oil is then collected by distillation.

Another processing method is to concentrate the Ginger oil and this is made commercially by using solvents. The solvent evaporates leaving a thick paste that is used to flavor soft drinks.

ABOVE **Grate your own Ginger for maximum freshness**

TO MAKE A TINCTURE

STANDARD QUANTITY

Use 8oz (225g) of dried Ginger rhizome, shredded or powdered, or 11oz (310g) of fresh rhizome – grated or shredded – to 4 cups (1 liter) of alcohol and water mixture.

1 Put the Ginger in a liquidizer and cover with vodka; there is no need to liquidize powdered Ginger – simply cover with vodka and stir well. You can use 45% proof vodka, but 70–80% proof is better. Blend the ingredients, then pour into a sterilized, airtight, dark glass jar. Shake well and store in a dark place.

2 After two days, measure the contents and add water. Add 20% of water to the total quantity if using standard vodka and 50–60% if using 70–80% proof vodka. Leave for at least two weeks and shake the jar daily.

3 Strain the tincture through a jelly-bag, preferably overnight. For best results, you can use a wine press. Pour into bottles and label. Store in a cool, dark place for up to two years. For personal use, decant into a 2fl oz (50ml) bottle. For dosages, see page 32.

TO MAKE GINGER BEER

STANDARD QUANTITY

1oz (25g) fresh Ginger rhizome to 18 cups (4.5 liters) water, 1 sliced lemon, 1 tsp cream of tartar, ½lb (225g) cane sugar, ½oz (15g) brewers' yeast, 1 egg white (or vegan alternative)

1 Bruise the Ginger and place it in a large saucepan with the water. Bring to a boil then simmer for 30 minutes.

2 Remove the Ginger and pour the liquid into a large bowl. Add the lemon (including the rind), cream of tartar, and sugar. Stir until the sugar has dissolved, then let cool.

3 When the liquid is lukewarm, stir in the yeast. Then cover the bowl with a clean cloth and leave to ferment for two days.

4 Skim off the scum and strain the beer into another bowl. Then whisk in the egg white and pour the mixture into sterilized glass bottles. For ginger beer, you must use thick bottles, preferably with screw-tops, because thin glass bottles have a tendency to explode. Keep for at least three weeks in a cupboard before drinking, then store in a refrigerator.

TINCTURES: RECOMMENDED DOSAGE

🌿 **Everyday use** *Adults: 1 tsp (5ml) diluted in about 5 tsp (25ml) of water, 2–5 times daily. Children: over 12 years, adult dose; 7–12 years, half adult dose; 3–7 years, quarter adult dose; younger than 3 years, consult a qualified herbalist.*

🌿 **Acute conditions** *Adults: 1 tsp (5ml), diluted as above, every ½ hour until severe symptoms subside. Children: over 12 years, adult dose; 7–12 years, ½ tsp (2.5ml); 3–7 years, ¼ tsp (1.25ml) every ½ hour; younger than 3 years, consult a herbalist.*

🌿 **Long term** *Adults: 1 tsp (5ml), diluted as above, 1–2 times daily for 2–3 months. Children: over 12 years, adult dose; 7–12 years, half adult dose; 3–7 years, quarter adult dose; younger than 3 years, consult a herbalist. With professional guidance, you may continue for longer periods.*

TINCTURES AND THE MOON'S PHASES

There is much lore associated with the harvesting and use of healing plants, and Ginger is no exception. Even today, many herbalists ensure that their medications are in phase with nature and advocate that the preparation of a tincture should coincide with the gravitational waxing and waning of the moon. If you would like to keep to this tradition, begin the process when the moon is new, then strain and bottle the Ginger tincture at the time of the full moon.

REMOVING THE ALCOHOL

If you prefer to avoid the small amount of alcohol that is found in herbal tinctures – especially important if you are pregnant or diabetic – add a little boiling water to your dose and leave it to stand for five minutes. In this way, approximately 98.5% of the alcohol will evaporate. If you need to avoid alcohol entirely, homemade tinctures can be prepared using a mixture of apple cider vinegar and water.

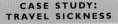
GINGER TINCTURE SYRUP

If you do not like the taste of Ginger, you can sweeten the standard tincture to make a syrup. Children in particular often prefer taking syrup to tincture. It is easy to make and will store for a month in the right conditions.

BELOW *Honey can make the tincture more palatable.*

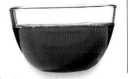

CASE STUDY: TRAVEL SICKNESS

Motion sickness was more than just a minor irritant for Amanda. She used to watch enviously as friends set off on exotic trips, but despite trying all the standard medications, she was so sick and miserable in planes, cars, and ships that she never went anywhere at all. A friend, who was a nurse, recommended that she try Ginger. The next weekend, Amanda took two capsules before setting off on a long car journey and then took two more every couple of hours. She hardly felt nauseous at all and was delighted. She now takes Ginger capsules with her on all car trips and has even managed to fly and sail.

TO MAKE GINGER TINCTURE SYRUP

STANDARD QUANTITY

1–4 parts tincture to 1–3 parts organic honey or maple syrup

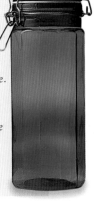

1 Mix one to four parts of tincture with one to three parts of cold-pressed, organic, runny honey or maple syrup in a sterilized, dark glass jar. The ingredients may be mixed to taste in a ratio as high as four parts tincture to one part honey (sweet) or one part tincture to one part honey (sweetest).

2 Label the jar clearly; keep in a cool, dark place. Shake the jar well before dispensing each dose.

Recommended dosage

Take as directed for tincture (see opposite), with extra volume to allow for added honey.

GINGER DECOCTION

Water-based processes preserve some of the many medicinal qualities of Ginger. A decoction, therefore, can be a useful way to prepare the rhizome. Dried Ginger may be used, but fresh ingredients (if available) are always best.

DECOCTION SYRUP

You can make this preparation in the same way as tincture syrup (see page 33), but use a decoction instead of a tincture. Take the same dose as given below for a decoction, but allow for the honey, if you have added a significant volume.

TO MAKE A DECOCTION

STANDARD QUANTITY

¾oz (20g) of dried or 1½oz (40g) of chopped fresh Ginger rhizome to 3 cups (750ml) of cold water. This reduces down to about 2 cups (500ml) of liquid after simmering – enough for about 2 cups

1 *Put the Ginger in a saucepan (a double boiler is ideal) with the water, and simmer on a very low heat for 20–30 minutes. During this time, the liquid should reduce by about a third. Leave to cool. Then strain into a pitcher.*

2 *Pour out a cup dose, then store the remainder in a cool place, or refrigerate if storing for longer than a day. For traveling, strain off the mixture while still hot into a thermos bottle to take with you.*

Recommended dosage
Adults: 2 cups daily – in total 2 cups (500ml) per day. Children: over 12 years, adult dose; 7–12 years, half adult dose; 3–7 years, quarter adult dose; under 3 years, a few sips at a time, totaling 6 tsp (30ml) a day.

GINGER INFUSION (TEA)

A cup of Ginger tea is a quick and effective method for improving the appetite, which can be of great benefit to those recovering from illnesses, especially those who may not feel like eating. Some people find that a tea (tisane) made with Ginger is beneficial in the treatment of various complaints connected with the digestive and urinary systems. In particular, Ginger tea aids the digestion by reducing internal gas.

It is best to use freshly grated rhizome, but you can use dried if fresh is unavailable. However, the powder can be a little too strong and the flavor not nearly so pleasant since it lacks some of the herb's essential oils.

TO MAKE AN INFUSION

STANDARD QUANTITY

2 tsp (4–6g) freshly grated Ginger rhizome or 1 tsp (5g) dried, powdered rhizome added to 1 cup (250ml) of water (makes 1 cup)

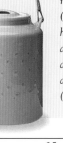

1 Put the Ginger in a tea sock and place in a cup or teapot. Pour on boiling water and let it infuse for 7–10 minutes.

2 Remove the tea sock and, if desired, add ½ tsp (2.5ml) of organic, cold-pressed honey.

NOTE

Teas can also be made in a teapot infuser, or in a coffee pot with a plunger.

Recommended dosage

Adults: 2 cups (500ml) daily for recovery from illness, or ½ cup (125ml) daily for general good health. Children: over 12 years, adult dose; 9–12 years, half adult dose; 1–9 years, quarter adult dose; younger than 1 year, 2 tsp (10ml) in total per day.

GINGER JUICE

In China, 1 tsp (5ml) each of Ginger juice and water is used as a gargle. If the throat is sore, you can add up to 1 cup (250ml) of water. The gargle is then swallowed. The process is repeated every four hours, to help eliminate toxins from the body.

For a detoxifying drink, mix Ginger juice with carrot or apple juice in a ratio of 1:19.

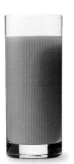

ABOVE *For a cleansing tonic, try Carrot and Ginger juice.*

RIGHT *Gargling with Ginger juice in water can help soothe and relieve a sore throat.*

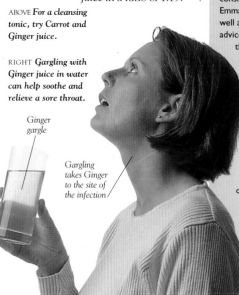

Ginger gargle

Gargling takes Ginger to the site of the infection

CASE STUDY: COLDS AND FLU

Emma had been asthmatic since early childhood. In her early twenties, she led a very busy lifestyle and often felt quite rundown and dispirited. In these situations, Emma was prone to colds, flu, and chest infections that brought on asthma attacks. She was eager to take more control over her health, rather than relying on the medications that had been prescribed for her, and began to consider alternative treatments. Emma consulted an herbalist who, as well as giving her diet and lifestyle advice, suggested taking Ginger in the form of decoctions – and occasionally tinctures for ease of use. Emma found it helped to alleviate some of the symptoms of her colds, especially any chills she suffered – it warmed her body and helped to lower fevers. More remarkably, Ginger's antibacterial actions helped to prevent infections from occurring altogether. Emma began to enjoy a higher standard of health, and her increased energy levels enabled her to join the local gym, thereby further increasing her stamina and enjoyment of life.

GINGER CAPSULES

Capsules can easily be made from powdered, dried Ginger. If preferred, capsules can be filled with root that is freshly grated using the finest holes on a cheese grater, but must be consumed immediately.

You can also buy powdered Ginger in capsule or tablet form. Capsules make an ideal portable remedy and suit those who dislike too much Ginger in their food.

Commercially produced capsules are available that contain a standardized amount of pharmaceutically active constituents from Ginger. Some companies give their capsules a high gingerol content, while others include Ginger's more pungent compounds. Consult an herbalist if you are not sure which capsules are best to buy for your condition.

TO MAKE CAPSULES

STANDARD QUANTITY

Approximately 250–300mg of powdered Ginger fits into a size 00 capsule. Gelatin-free capsules for vegetarians are also available.

1 *Put a little dried, finely powdered Ginger in a saucer and separate the two halves of the capsule.*

2 *Using the capsule ends as shovels, push them together until each end is full (one end will be less so), then carefully slide them together.*

Recommended dosage

Adults: 1–2 capsules 1–3 times daily. Children: over 12 years, adult dose; 7–12 years, half adult dose. Ginger capsules are generally not given to children under 7. Ginger tea would be more suitable or give fresh Ginger in food. Alternatively, you could mix ¼ tsp of Ginger powder with stiff honey and give it in small amounts throughout the day.

RIGHT *Scoop the powdered herb into each end of a capsule.*

Preparations for external use

GINGER FORMS THE BASE *for many external treatments for strains, sprains, muscle aches and pains, and poor circulation. It has been used in this way for centuries and there are a variety of external preparations from ointments to poultices that may be made with Ginger.*

ABOVE **Ginger ointment** *helps relieve stiffness.*

Although it may be best known for its internal applications, Ginger is a fine herb for treating a number of external complaints. For best results take it internally at the same time, in the form of an infusion, in order to reinforce the action of the plant.

GINGER BATH

For people with arthritis, a tendency to chilblains, and, of course, those with sprains or widespread muscular aches or strains, 2 cups (500ml) of Ginger decoction, or Ginger Water (see right), can be added to a shallow bath to bring relief from discomfort.

GINGER OINTMENT

Ointments are semi-solid preparations that protect and nourish the skin and bring medication to the underlying tissues. Ginger ointment is ideal

TO MAKE GINGER WATER

STANDARD QUANTITY

2 cups (200g) freshly grated Ginger, 10½fl oz (300ml) distilled water, a small, thinly pared piece of orange rind

1 *Mix the Ginger, water, and orange rind in a small, heatproof, enamel or glass pan. Cover, and bring to a boil.*

2 *Simmer for 10 minutes. Remove from the heat, and let infuse for 1–2 hours or overnight.*

CASE STUDY: SPORTS INJURY

In the last few months Martin, an avid sportsman, had sprained his knee and suffered a number of muscle strains. Each time he had used ice packs to reduce the swelling and pain, but recovery was always slow. A friend suggested rubbing a Ginger-based ointment into the affected area and Martin was surprised by the warming, soothing effect that it provided. Protective bandaging of the knee before taking part in any training helped to prevent a recurrence of his knee injuries.

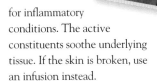

for inflammatory conditions. The active constituents soothe underlying tissue. If the skin is broken, use an infusion instead.

3 Strain the liquid, pressing the Ginger and orange peel against the sieve to extract the fragrant oil. Bottle in sterilized, dark glass jars and label carefully. The Ginger water will last for 3 days in the refrigerator. It can be used as a hot (when reheated) or cold compress to help heal bruises and inflammation, and as a skin cleanser.

TO MAKE AN OINTMENT

STANDARD QUANTITY

12fl oz (350ml) of olive oil, 11oz (300g) of powdered Ginger, 2oz (50g) beeswax

1 Mix the olive oil and Ginger in a closed container. Either put in an oven – heated to approximately 100°F (38°C) – for an hour, or stand in the sun for a week.

2 If using the oven method, leave for a further week to macerate and then heat again before straining. Strain through a large colander lined with a piece of cheesecloth.

3 Melt the beeswax in a double boiler or saucepan with a thick base, over a very low heat, and add the herbal olive oil mixture. Have sterilized, dark glass jars ready. Put a little of the liquid into one of them to check that it is the correct consistency for use. Fill the jars and label clearly.

LEFT **Ginger water makes a good facial cleanser.**

39

GINGER COMPRESS

One of the principal substances used as a base for various treatments for sprained joints, muscular strains, and fibrositis, Ginger is also employed for the relief of rheumatoid arthritis and osteoarthritis. A compress made with Ginger directly and quickly brings comfort to such conditions through its anti-inflammatory and pain-relieving actions. It is also invaluable for indigestion, liver, kidney, and gallstone inflammation, and menstrual cramps. Applying a hot-water bottle can speed up the process.

GINGER POULTICE

A poultice is an ideal treatment for a swollen knee or an aching leg. Freshly grated or powdered Ginger can be added to a cooked, mashed potato and, while still warm, spread over the affected area. It can be left on for 2 hours or overnight. The heat generated helps Ginger's active constituents to travel quickly to the affected area, where pain and swelling will be alleviated.

RIGHT *Fresh Ginger for a poultice.*

TO MAKE A COMPRESS

STANDARD QUANTITY

10½fl oz (300 ml) Ginger decoction (see page 34) or enough chopped fresh Ginger to cover the affected part

1 *Either cover the knee with chopped fresh Ginger or with a piece of cheesecloth soaked in warm Ginger decoction. Secure it firmly in place with plenty of plastic wrap.*

2 *Leave for 10–20 minutes and then repeat. The compress may be reapplied two or three times, with the last one being left in position for 1–2 hours.*

LEFT *A compress made with fresh Ginger (right) eases knee pain.*

To make the poultice, cook and mash one large potato. Then add 1 tbsp of freshly grated Ginger rhizome, or 3 tsp dried and powdered, and mix together into a paste. While it is still warm, apply it to the area, then secure it firmly in place with a bandage or plastic wrap.

OTHER APPLICATIONS

Mouthwash and gargle

A powerful mouthwash can be made by diluting 2 tsp (10ml) of Ginger tincture in half a glass of water. Although the taste is quite strong, this solution will help to stop infections of the gums, mucous membranes, and throat. Gargling with the same mixture is effective in the treatment of sore throats (see page 36).

BELOW *Massage with Ginger oil relaxes the muscles and improves the circulation.*

Soothing pressure

Oils penetrate the skin

Massage oil

Ginger is very useful in massage when combined with a base oil. To make 1 cup (250ml) of base oil, mix ½ cup (150ml) sunflower oil with 2fl oz (50ml) each of olive oil and almond oil. Then add about 1 tsp (4–6ml) of Ginger essential oil – the exact amount depends on strength required. This can be used to make a stimulating massage oil, which smells wonderful. Alternatively, combine 1 cup (250ml) of the base oil with ½ tsp (2ml) Ginger, and ¼ tsp (1ml) each of Rosemary, Chamomile, and Black Pepper essential oils. Apply a few drops to a small area before using it on the whole body; avoid using it on the face; and never apply neat essential oil to the skin.

CAUTION

Do not use this massage oil if you are pregnant or breastfeeding.

Natural medicine for everyone

GINGER IS GENERALLY SAFE, *and clinical trials have shown that side-effects are very rare.*

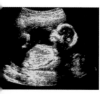

ABOVE *A safe herb, Ginger does not harm the developing fetus.*

PREGNANCY

Because of its known effects upon the sex hormones, some people advise that Ginger should be used with caution during pregnancy (see page 21). However, there have been no recorded cases of Ginger inducing uterine contractions or miscarriages. In fact it is a traditional remedy for morning sickness, bringing great relief to many women.

CAUTION

There are a few instances when Ginger should be avoided. For example, it should not be taken by people with "heated" liver conditions, such as hepatitis, where further heat would not be wise. Some conditions where the kidneys become hot and inflamed should also not be further exacerbated by Ginger. If you are in any doubt, consult a medical herbalist before taking Ginger.

CHILDREN

There are few children's medicines that contain Ginger. The taste of this spice is pleasant, however, and the herb may be used to stimulate the appetite and ease digestive problems and nausea. Ginger has the advantage with children of being available in a number of tempting forms, including syrup, Ginger beer, and crystallized Ginger. If a child over 7 years does not like the taste, try giving capsules, which are very useful for travel sickness – a common children's complaint.

RIGHT *Ginger is an ideal remedy for common childhood complaints such as indigestion and nausea.*

ELDERLY PEOPLE

Ginger has a number of useful applications for elderly people. For example, it helps to prevent blood clot formation and has an important role in the prevention of heart attacks and strokes in people known to be susceptible. Ginger's stimulating effect upon the circulatory system is ideal for helping to keep the elderly warm, and its powerful anti-inflammatory action is of great benefit to many people who suffer from rheumatoid arthritis or osteoarthritis.

The elderly also often have problems with digestion and here again Ginger will help.

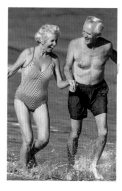

LEFT *Elderly people will find Ginger warming and stimulating.*

CAUTION

It is normally safe to take Ginger alongside other prescription medicines, but check with your herbalist or doctor first, especially if you are pregnant, have a serious illness such as cancer, suffer from gastrointestinal complaints including ulcers, or have a liver or kidney condition.

CASE STUDY: PERIOD PAINS

Sandra dreaded glancing at the calendar because every month her period pains were awful. In particular she disliked the pelvic and abdominal cramps that seemed to consume her entire being in a rhythmic cycle of pain. Eventually, she went to a herbal practitioner who prescribed Ginger in the form of a tincture as part of a composite formula. Its antispasmodic properties went right to work, relaxing the muscles in her pelvic region and helping to relieve the cramping pains by encouraging better circulation.

Sandra soon learned that she could take Ginger in different ways, so when her periods began, she would drink warming Ginger teas, or suck on candied Ginger when she was too busy to sit down for a hot drink. If the cramps threatened to be very strong, a warm Ginger compress applied to her stomach was particularly soothing and relaxing. Now Sandra is no longer anxious about her periods.

Herbal combinations

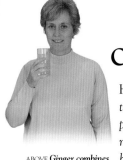

ABOVE **Ginger combines well with other herbs.**

HERBAL COMBINATIONS ARE USED *to complement the effect of a single herb. However, if you are pregnant or breastfeeding, or if you have a serious medical condition, consult your doctor or qualified herbalist first.*

Medicinal formulas often consist of several herbs with different, but complementary, actions. It is not unusual for such treatments to consist of one main herb with one or two others added to support its action and to address different underlying causes of the ailment. For example, to treat a fever, Ginger may be suggested in order to promote perspiration and thereby reduce the temperature, with additional herbs to help fight infection and to ensure a good night's sleep.

RIGHT **Take warming herbal remedies to relieve chilblains.**

POOR CIRCULATION

Ginger is a hot spice with a stimulating, decongestive action in the body. This tincture formula is ideal for people who suffer from cold hands and feet, especially if it results in conditions such as chilblains.

Formula 1 part Ginger rhizome, 2 parts Hawthorn berries, 2 parts Prickly Ash bark.

Dosage Adults: 1 tsp (5ml) tincture 3–4 times daily. Children: consult a doctor or herbalist.

CAUTION

Do not take Prickly Ash in pregnancy.

In this combination, Ginger is a warming constituent.

The Hawthorn berries are able to strengthen the cardiac muscle and increase the blood flow through the heart without raising its rate or the blood pressure. In this way, circulation is improved to the peripheral capillaries.

Prickly Ash bark stimulates the circulation in the peripheral capillaries.

The overall effect of this formula is to warm and enliven both mind and body.

COLDS AND CHEST INFECTIONS

Taken as a warm decoction, this combination of Ginger, Saw Palmetto, Echinacea, and Eucalyptus will act upon the respiratory system, helping to keep the tract clear from catarrh, as well as fighting infection.

Formula 1 part Ginger rhizome, 2 parts Saw Palmetto berries, 2 parts Echinacea root, 1 part Eucalyptus leaves.

Dosage Adults: 5fl oz (150ml) decoction 3 times daily. Children: over 12 years, adult dose; 7–12 years, half adult dose; under 7 years, consult a professional herbalist.

Saw Palmetto berries

In this decoction, Ginger reduces the effects of chills, lowers fever, and helps to reduce the likelihood of further colds.

Saw Palmetto berries are useful for their action as an expectorant, helping to reduce congestion from phlegm.

Echinacea was considered by the Native Americans to be a "sacred herb." It increases the general effectiveness of the immune system and particularly stimulates the infection-fighting activity of white blood cells.

The distinctive aroma of Eucalyptus leaves provides the drink with a clean, fresh taste and helps to clear the lungs and open the sinuses, bringing relief from any congestion.

Echinacea root

Eucalyptus leaves

COLITIS AND DIVERTICULITIS

There are a number of conditions in which inflammation of the digestive system is present, and the following combination of tinctures is particularly helpful in the treatment of colitis, diverticulitis, and "leaky gut" (see page 57). It is also important to follow a balanced diet for these illnesses and to avoid foods that may be causing an allergic reaction.

Formula 1 part Ginger rhizome, 3 parts Wild Yam root, 2 parts Chamomile flowers, 1 part Marshmallow root.

Dosage Adults: 1 tsp (5ml) of tincture 3–4 times daily. Children: over 12 years, adult dose; 7–12 years, half adult dose. Under 7 years, consult a professional herbalist.

Ginger helps reduce intestinal gas and discomfort, and also has an anti-inflammatory effect.

Marshmallow root

The Wild Yam in the remedy acts upon the body in many ways that are similar to Ginger. It is known as "colic root" and works as a muscle relaxant, thereby reducing cramps. It is of particular benefit in the treatment of diverticulitis.

Chamomile is a relaxant and mild sedative. It reduces tension and does not have unpleasant side effects. It also has a localized anti-inflammatory effect.

Marshmallow root is a soothing herb known to affect the digestive system beneficially by lining and protecting the wall of the stomach and bowel – helping to soothe and heal the mucous membranes and tissues in the process.

Dried Chamo flowers

RIGHT **A remedy based on Ginger can soothe away digestive problems.**

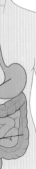

oesophagus

stomach

colon

RIGHT **The Chinese use sliced, dried Ginger medicinally.**

PAINFUL MENSTRUATION

Although Ginger makes a significant contribution toward reducing menstrual cramps when taken on its own, some women require a little extra help. This combination of herbal tinctures is a particularly powerful all-round remedy for period pain.

Ginger rhizome

Formula 2 parts Ginger rhizome, 1 part Black Cohosh bark, 2 parts Cramp bark, 1 part Valerian root.

Dosage Adults: 1 tsp (5ml) of tincture 3–4 times 1–2 days prior to menstruation.

Ginger is a powerful herb that reduces menstrual cramps by helping to relax the smooth muscle in the pelvic region.

Black Cohosh bark is also antispasmodic and has a balancing action on the hormones. It allows rigid muscles to relax and assists inert muscles in working more effectively.

Cramp bark is specifically useful for muscular cramps and pains in the abdominal region, especially in the uterus.

Valerian root relaxes the nervous system and helps to calm the whole body.

In general, this formula relaxes the whole pelvic region, helping to ensure a balanced menstrual flow. It also relieves pain and discomfort.

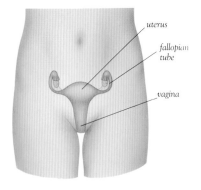

uterus

fallopian tube

vagina

ABOVE **Tense uterine muscles may be relaxed with antispasmodic herbs.**

Valerian root

CAUTION

Do not take Valerian with other sleep-inducing drugs.

LEFT **Cramp bark relieves period pain.**

WEIGHT LOSS AND ASSOCIATED NAUSEA

Ginger has an important role to play in illnesses where there is weight loss due to loss of appetite. This mixture of herbal tinctures combines Ginger with other digestive herbs.

Formula 2 parts each of Ginger rhizome, Saw Palmetto berries, Schisandra berries, Fenugreek seeds, and 1 part Gentian root.

Dosage Adults: 1 tsp (5ml) of tincture 3–4 times daily. Children: over 12 adult dose; 7–12 years, half adult dose; under 7 years, you should consult a doctor or qualified herbalist.

Schisandra berries

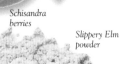

Slippery Elm powder

Gentian root

> ### CAUTION
>
> Do not take Fenugreek in pregnancy or Gentian if you have a peptic ulcer.

Ginger relieves nausea associated with lack of appetite. It stimulates saliva and digestive juices, and encourages the appetite. It will also help to process food without indigestion.

Saw Palmetto has a marked effect upon tissue, helping to build strength and body mass quickly. It also stimulates appetite and assists digestion.

Schisandra berries, which in Chinese medicine are considered to taste of all five elemental energies, stimulate the appetite and are a fine tonic herb. The European digestive herb, Gentian, encourages the release of bile and supports the entire digestive system, especially the liver.

Additionally, adults may take 2 tsp (10ml) of Slippery Elm powder 3 times daily. Put the powder in a sterilized jar, add 1 cup (250ml) of water, shake and drink immediately. There is no quicker way to build up the body.

TRAVEL SICKNESS AND NAUSEA

Ginger can quell motion sickness and is supported in medical literature as an alternative to prescribed medicines.

Formula 2 parts each of Ginger rhizome, Peppermint leaf, and Angelica root, and 1 part Chamomile flowers.

Dosage Adults: 1 tsp (5ml) of tincture 3–4 times daily. Children: over 12 years, adult dose; 7–12 years, half adult dose; 3–7 years, quarter adult dose; under 3 years, consult an herbalist.

Ginger is the principal anti-emetic agent in this formula, but Peppermint is also antiemetic and eases diarrhea, indigestion, cramps, and nausea.

The Angelica and Chamomile complete this powerful formula for dealing with upset stomachs.

BELOW *Ginger and Peppermint are traditional remedies for travel sickness.*

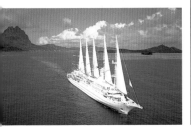

CONSTIPATION

This formula, combined with plenty of exercise, can bring relief from constipation.

Formula 2 parts Ginger rhizome, 2 parts Rhubarb root (*Rumex crispus*), 2 parts Barberry root bark, 1 part Cascara bark.

Dosage Adults: 1 tsp (5ml) of tincture 1–3 times daily. Children: over 12 years, adult dose; 7–12 years, half adult dose; 3–7 years, quarter adult dose; under 3 years, consult a doctor or qualified herbalist.

Ginger helps elimination and eases the pains of colic.

Rhubarb aids digestion and evacuation, while Barberry stimulates the digestive system.

Cascara activates a sluggish bowel, speeding up evacuation.

ABOVE *Brisk exercise keeps the digestive tract healthy.*

CAUTION

Do not take Rhubarb and Barberry in pregnancy. Omit Cascara if constipation is mild, and do not exceed the stated dose because it can cause dehydration.

How Ginger works

GINGER'S USE *all over the world for hundreds of years has given us a wealth of understanding about its beneficial properties – knowledge that is now backed up by recent research studies.*

$$CH_3O \qquad\qquad O \qquad OH$$
$$\qquad\qquad\qquad (CH_2)_4CH_3$$
$$HO$$

ABOVE **Gingerol helps prevent vomiting.**

Scientists have analyzed the chemical composition of Ginger and found it contains a wide variety of chemical substances.

The effects of Ginger's active constituents are well known. Cumene, for example, has a narcotic effect, and the volatile oil (made up of borneol, cineole, citral, mucilage, phellandrene, resin, starch, zingiberene, and zingiberole) stimulates the circulation and causes sweating. The resin contains the important gingerol and shogaol, and is known to inhibit the manufacture of prostaglandins (which act as local hormones), thereby warming the body and assisting circulation. Gingerol helps block the action of the chemical messenger serotonin, which makes the stomach contract to cause vomiting.

The effects of other constituents, however, have yet to be established. For example, Ginger is known to prevent food from oxidizing (going brown) so it is possible that it may also act internally to prevent the oxidation, that leads to the development of harmful free radicals (see page 57). This may help to explain how the intake of Ginger leads to a lower cholesterol level, since it is known that cholesterol is more easily removed from the body if it has not been oxidized.

LEFT **Ginger contains literally hundreds of active constituents.**

MAIN EFFECTS

The principal actions of Ginger can be traced back to the qualities of its individual chemical constituents. The herb:
* stimulates the body's systems;
* interferes with the blood-clotting mechanism;
* acts as an anti-inflammatory, reducing pain and discomfort;
* is a powerful antiemetic, especially effective for nausea after surgery and motion sickness.

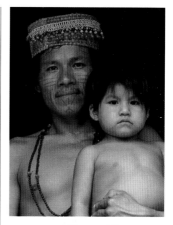

ABOVE *The use of Ginger by Amazonian tribes is stimulating research.*

RECENT STUDIES

Scientific studies into the effects of Ginger include the antiplatelet effects of one of Ginger's main chemical components – gingerol; the antiemetic uses of Ginger post-operatively; the molluscicidal and antischistosomal activities of Ginger (see page 58).

RESEARCH

More research is needed to investigate the range of traditional uses for Ginger. Amazonian tribes, for example, use it to relieve stomach aches, headaches, and diarrhea, and employ its leaves as a compress to relieve pain.

It has recently been shown that Ginger is able to reduce vertigo as well as nausea, while a study at St. Bartholomew's Hospital, London, suggested the herb was more useful than conventional antiemetics for nausea after surgery.

In Shandong, China, a paste of raw Ginger and brown sugar cured 70% of a group of 50 patients with bacterial dysentery in under five days.

In the future, scientific research may endorse many more medicinal uses for this outstanding herb.

Conditions chart

THIS CHART *is a guide to some of the ailments that Ginger can treat, but it is not intended to replace other forms of treatment. Always consult your doctor or other qualified medical practitioner before embarking on a course of treatment. Follow dosages and application guidance given earlier in this book unless otherwise stated.*

NAME	INTERNAL USE	EXTERNAL USE
ANGINA	Decoction, tea, tincture, capsule	
BLOOD CLOTS	Decoction, tea, tincture, capsule	
CHILBLAINS	Tincture, capsule, Ginger water	Ointment
CIRCULATORY DISORDERS	Decoction, tincture, tea, capsule, syrup	
COLIC	Decoction, tincture, tea, capsule, syrup	
CONSTIPATION	Decoction, tincture, tea, capsule, syrup	
COUGH	Tincture, tea, capsule, syrup, gargle	

NAME	INTERNAL USE	EXTERNAL USE
DIGESTIVE DISORDERS	Decoction, tincture, tea, capsule, syrup	
DYSPEPSIA	Decoction, tincture, tea, capsule, syrup	
FEVER	Decoction, tincture, tea, capsule, syrup	
FIBROSITIS	Tincture, capsule compress, poultice	Ointment
FLATULENCE	Tincture, tea, capsule	
INDIGESTION	Tincture, tea, capsule	
INFLUENZA	Tincture, tea, capsule	
JOINT SPRAIN	Tincture, capsule, Ginger water	Ointment, compress, poultice, massage oil
"LEAKY GUT" (DYSBIOSIS)	Decoction, tincture, tea, capsule, syrup	

NAME	INTERNAL USE	EXTERNAL USE
MENSTRUAL CRAMPS	Decoction, tincture, tea, capsule	
MENSTRUATION (PAINFUL)	Decoction, tincture, tea, capsule	Compress, massage oil
MORNING SICKNESS	Decoction, tincture, tea, capsule, syrup	
MOTION SICKNESS	Decoction, tincture, tea, capsule, syrup	
MUCUS CONGESTION	Decoction, tincture, tea, capsule, syrup	
MUSCLE STRAIN	Decoction, tincture, tea, capsule, syrup, Ginger water	Massage oil, poultice
MUSCULAR ACHES AND PAINS	Decoction, tincture, tea, capsule, syrup, Ginger water	Massage oil, poultice
NAUSEA	Decoction, tincture, tea, capsule, syrup	
OSTEOARTHRITIS	Decoction, tincture, tea, capsule, syrup	Compress, massage oil
PAINFUL PERIODS	Tincture, capsule	
POOR CIRCULATION	Tincture, capsule	

NAME	INTERNAL USE	EXTERNAL USE
PARASITES	Decoction, tincture, tea, capsule	
RHEUMATOID ARTHRITIS	Tincture, capsule	Ointment, compress
SCHISTOSOMIASIS (BILHARZIA)	Decoction, tincture, tea, capsule, syrup	
SORE THROAT	Decoction, tincture, tea, capsule, syrup, gargle	
SWOLLEN JOINT	Decoction, tincture, tea, capsule, syrup	Compress, massage oil
TOXINS	Decoction, tincture, tea, capsule, syrup, juice, gargle	
TRAVEL SICKNESS	Decoction, tincture, tea, capsule, syrup	
WIND (FLATULENCE)	Decoction, tincture, tea, capsule, syrup	

Glossary

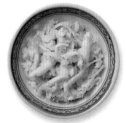
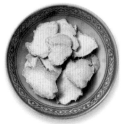
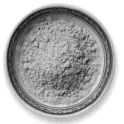

ANAPHYLAXIS
An extreme allergic reaction to a particular substance.

ANTIBACTERIAL
The ability of a substance to destroy or inhibit the growth of bacteria.

ANTIEMETIC
A substance that helps to prevent nausea and vomiting.

ANTI-INFLAMMATORY
Reduces inflammation.

ANTIOXIDANT
Prevents oxidation. Protects against free radicals that cause cancer.

CASCADE EFFECT
A complex sequence of biochemical reactions resulting in the clotting of blood.

DERMATITIS
Inflammation of the skin.

DECOCTION
Method of preparing and preserving herbs in water.

EXPECTORANT
Substance that promotes the elimination of mucus from the respiratory tract.

FIBROSITIS
Condition characterized by inflammation of connective tissue.

FREE RADICALS
Highly reactive particles that damage cell membranes, DNA, and other cellular structures.

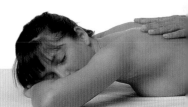

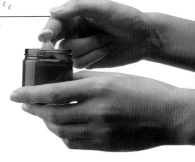

INFUSION
A herbal tea used for medicinal purposes. It may be drunk hot or cold.

LEAKY GUT
A condition where the stomach becomes porous: it is no longer a "sealed unit" and allows toxins to leak into the bloodstream.

NAUSEA
A feeling of sickness with an inclination to vomit.

PLATELETS
Disk-shaped fragments enclosed in cell membranes that flow through the blood and promote clotting.

STIMULANT
A substance that promotes increased activity in a function or system of the body.

SYNERGIST
A drug that interacts with another to produce greater effects than can be produced by each drug on its own.

TINCTURE
Plant medicine prepared by soaking herbs in alcohol and water.

TISANE
A herbal infusion or tea.

TONIC
A health-promoting substance inducing feelings of vigor.

TOPICAL
A treatment that is applied to the surface of the body as opposed to being taken internally.

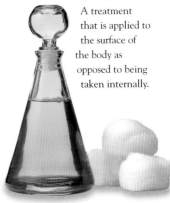

Bibliography

"ANTI-PLATELET EFFECT OF GINGEROL ISOLATED FROM ZINGIBER OFFICINALE," *Jih-Hwa Guh, et al.* (Pharm. Pharmacol., 47: 329-332, 1995)

BARTRAM'S ENCYCLOPEDIA OF HERBAL MEDICINE, *Thomas Bartram* (Robinson, 1998)

"CHINA NUMBER ONE GINGER," (www.thespicehouse.com/chinanumb eroneginger.htm, 29 April 1999)

THE COMPLETE ILLUSTRATED HOLISTIC HERBAL, *David Hoffmann* (Element Books, 1996)

THE ENCYCLOPEDIA OF MEDICINAL PLANTS, *Andrew Chevallier* (Dorling Kindersley, 1996)

THE ESSENTIAL BOOK OF HERBAL MEDICINE, *Simon Y. Mills* (Arkana, 1993)

GINGER: COMMON SPICE AND WONDER DRUG, *Paul Shulick* (Herbal Free Press, 1996)

GINGER: THE ULTIMATE HOME REMEDY, *Dr. Stephen Fulder* (Souvenir Press, 1993)

"GINGER, PART I," *Mary Conley* (www.accessnewage.com/articles/heal th/ginger1.htm, 1999)

"GINGER, PART II," *Mary Conley* (www.accessnewage.com/articles/heal th/ginger2.htm, 1999)

HERBAL GIFTS, *Jane Newdick* (CLB, 1999)

HERBALGRAM, the Journal of the American Botanical Council and the Herb Research Foundation

HERBAL HEALING FOR WOMEN, *Rosemary Gladstar* (Bantam Books, 1994)

THE HERB SOCIETY'S HOME HERBAL, *Penelope Ody* (Dorling Kindersley, 1995)

THE HOLISTIC HERBAL, *David Hoffmann* (Element Books, 1988)

NATURE'S PHARMACY, *Christine Stockwell* (Century, 1988)

"INHIBITION OF TUMOR PROMOTION IN SENCAR MOUSE SKIN BY ETHANOL EXTRACT OF ZINGIBER OFFICINALE RHIZOME," *S. K. Katiyar et al.* (Cancer Research, 1996)

A MODERN HERBAL, *Mrs. M. Grieve* (Tiger Books, 1992)

"MOLLUSCICIDAL AND ANTISCHISTOSOMAL ACTIVITIES OF ZINGIBER OFFICINALE," *C. O. Adewunmi, et al.* (Planta Med. 1990)

POTTER'S NEW CYCLOPAEDIA OF BOTANICAL DRUGS AND PREPARATIONS *R. C. Wren* (Health Science Press, 1973)

ROMAN GARDENS AND THEIR PLANTS, *Claire Ryley* (Fishbourne Roman Palace, 1996)

THE COMPLETE BOOK OF HERBS, *Lesley Bremness* (Dorling Kindersley, 1988)

"ZINGIBER OFFICINALE (GINGER) – AN ANTIEMETIC FOR DAY CASE SURGERY," *S. Phillips, et al.* (Anaesthesia, 1993)

Useful addresses

ASSOCIATIONS AND SOCIETIES

**British Herbal Medicine
Association (B.H.M.A.)**
Sun House, Church Street, Stroud,
Glos. GL5 1JL, UK
Tel: 011 44 1453–751389
Fax: 011 44 1453–751402
Works with the Medicine Control
Agency to promote high standards of
quality and safety of herbal medicine

Herb Society
Deddington Hill Farm,
Warmington, Banbury,
Oxon OX17 1XB, UK
Tel: 011 44 1295–692000
Fax: 011 44 1295–692004
Educational charity that disseminates
information about herbs and
organizes workshops

**The Wild Plant Conservation
Charity**
The Natural History Museum,
Cromwell Road,
London SW7 5BD, UK
Tel: 011 44 171–938 9123
Registered charity to save British
wild plants

SUPPLIERS IN THE UK

Baldwin & Company
171–173 Walworth Road,
London SE17 1RW, UK
Tel: 011 44 171–703 5550
Herbs, storage bottles, jars, and
containers available

Hambleden Herbs
Court Farm, Milverton,
Somerset TA4 1NF, UK
Tel: 011 44 1823–401205
Organic herbs by mail order

Herbs, Hands, Healing
The Cabins, Station Warehouse,
Station Road, Pulham Market,
Norfolk IP21 4XF, UK
Tel/fax: 011 44 1379–608201
Organic herbal formulas &
Superfood; mail order; free brochure

SUPPLIERS/SCHOOLS IN THE USA

American Botanical Pharmacy
PO Box 3027, Santa Monica,
CA 90408, USA
Tel/fax: 1310 453–1987
Manufacturer and distributor of
herbal products; runs training courses

Blessed Herbs
109 Barre Plains Road,
Oakham,
MA 01068, USA
Tel: 1800 489–4372
Dried bulk herbs are available by
mail order in order to make your
own preparations

Stokes Tropicals
PO Box 9868, New Iberia,
LA 70562, USA
Tel: 1318 365 6998
Fax: 1318 365 6991
Web site: www.stokestropicals.com
Suppliers of all types of Ginger.